RESPIRATORY
&
ENT

OUTLINES for
MRCPCH

Dr Haitham Hassabou

ISBN: 9781672090476
ASIN: B082DYFSQ4

DEDICATED TO
MY FAMILY

CONTENTS

ACKNOWLEDGMENTS

I would like to thank my wife Alaa Nasr El-din, I am greatful to you , during stressful times , such as those faced when preparing for this book series . your advice continues to guide me , you where there when my thoughts dried ,you helped me calm down ,you did everything you could , I owe my everything to you .

Dr . Haitham Hassabou

1 - BRONCHIAL ASTHMA

- Hyperreactivity of airway to variety of stimuli .
- High degree of reversibility of obstruction either spontaneous or with treatment .

patterns of ashma

Viral Induced Wheeza	Classic Atopic Asthma (Multiple Trigger Asthma)	Cough Variant Asthma (Nocturnal Asthma)
-occur during winter with history of bronchiolitis in first year of life .	-occur due to release of mediators of inflammation from mast cell degranulation	-due to exposure to allergens in bed room
-with cold symptoms only	-triggered not only by colds but also non viral triggers as exercise or allergen s or smoke and cold air	-no colds
-symptoms free interval	-day to day symptoms	-nocturnal symptoms
-no family history of atopy	-positive FH of asthma -personal history of atopy -if both not present ..so the child mostly will outgrow asthma	-positive FH of atopy -personal history of atopy
-normal igE	-increase igE	
-poor response to regular anti inflammatory therapy	-resond well to regular anti inflammatory drugs	

1

Relieve Therapy		
-SABA	- SABA	-trial of SABA via spacer. -if failure to respond to SABA not exclude diagnosis But -another trial of ICS 4weeks Or two weeks of oral prednisolone
Prevention Therapy		
-if frequent or severe: Montelokast in winter time	-first line ICS	
Diagnosis		
-wheezy chest only during viral infection -atypical viral induced wheeze : **If** abrupt onset with poor response to bronchodilator ,suspecting the diagnosis of foreign body inhalation	**-more than one of** : nocturnal cough,dry or early morning, not moist cough -widespread wheeze -difficult breathing -chest tightness (**fop**)	-exercise induced cough and exercise intolerance -nocturnal cough -nevere wheeze -**diagnosis** done by spirometry or serial PEFR measurement in older age .(**FOP**)
-resolve by six years		

but can continue or change into multiple trigger wheeze	**Asthma predictive index: (AKP)** **Major criteria :** -parent history of asthma -personal atopic dermatitis **Minor criteria :** -blood osinophila >4 % -wheeze unrelated to cold -allergic rhinitis **One major or at least two minor** ,so it is more likely that asthma will persist .	
	Differential Diagnosis	

	-Mediastinal syndrome
	
	-Cystic fibrosis
	
	-Primary ciliary dyskinesia
	
	-Habitual cough **(FOP)**
	
	   o loud ,explosive and dry cough
	   o occur during day only
		-Allergic rhinitis
		
		-Adeniod s
		
		-Chronic sinusitis
		
		-Gerd

	- abscent at night	

Exercise Induced Asthma (EIA)

- Not specific variety of asthma.
- It is Sign of poor control in treated patient
- It may be the only manifestation of bronchial asthma
- Positive Family history of asthma
- Exercise induced cough =may be the only sign of exercise induced asthma
- It may persist for over two hours after exercise cessation.

Clinical Picture:

- Cough and wheezy chest several minutes after exercise
- Symptoms Increased by
  o   Cooling airway
  o   Running
  o   Cycling in cold
  o   Swimming
  so   warmup exercise is helpful

Diagnosis :

- No symptoms from other triggers, so it is not persistent asthma ,so no need for daily ICS.
- Normal baseline spirometry .
- Serial PEFR : variability more than 20%over weeks (**fop)**

Treatment :

- Preexercise inhaled Bronchodilator
  SABA via spacer before exercise (first line management)(**FOP)**

Differential Diagnosis :
- Vocal cord dysfunction (exercise induced dyspnea) see later

Management Of Asthma

- Asthma exacerbation

  - Progressive increase in more than one of : cough , wheeze,difficult breathing and chest tightness with low PEFR.
  - **Risk factors** : upper respiratory tract infection ,exposure to inhaled allergen ,poorly controlled asthma .
  - It is Severe asthma in emergency room
  - It is most common reason for admission
  - Typically hyperexpansion of lung in chest xray not indicate severity

- Assess severity of asthma : **(AKP)**

Mild Exacerbation	Moderate Exacerbation	Severe Exacerbation	Life Threating Asthma
Symptoms			
		Agitation , fatigue , only say 1-2 words ,may be abdominal pain , wheeze may be abscent (silent chest)	Drowsiness, confusion
Signs			
Saturation>92%	Saturation>92%	Saturation >90%	Saturation < 90%
		Tachycardia tachypnea	Bradypnea Cyanosis
		Pulsus paradoxicus <20	
		Marked retraction	

			Additional respiratory acidosis,impending respiratory failure
			Po2<8 kpa
PEFR in green zone 50-100%	PEFR in green zone 50-100%	PEFR in yellow zone 33-50 % performed in >= 8 years	PEFR<33%(red zone)
Treatment			
-No Oxygen	-No Oxygen	-High flow O2 via mask : Oxygen Not mandatory but only to maintain SO2 >92%	-High flow Oxygen via mask
Good response to salbutamol +- ipratropium bromide	Partial response to salbutamol+- ipratropium bromide		
Inhaler via **large volume spacer** +mask 10 puff /20 min for ist hr (if >20 kg) 5 puff /20 min for ist hr (if <20kg) Puff=100mcg	Inhaler via **large volume spacer** +mask	**-neublized B 2** agonists: Every 20min for one hour: 2.5 mg <5yr 5mg >= 5yr -add ipratropium bromide if no improvement after	Iv salbutomol **(AKP)**

		first neublized B2 agonists /20min **Dose:** ,25mg <12 year, 5mg >12 year **If stay confused with silent chest after half an hour** ,so intubation and iv salbutomol	
Then regular inhaler for 12 hrs or longer If deteriorate via neublizer As before	If deteriorate via neublizer As before		
Steriods : -prednisolone if no quick response -Home treatment when the patient improved .	Steriods : -prednisolone if no quick response **If improved** home treatment **If not improved** hospital admission	Steriods : -oral prednisolone -iv hydrocortisone Methyleprednisolone **Dose of prednisolone :** 20mg for 2-5 years 30-40mg for > 5yrs Weaning unneccessary unless exceed 14 days	**Intubation** if -Impaired oxygenation -Impaired ventilation = -Impending respiratory failure: -CO_2 >45 -Actual CO_2 more than expected CO_2
		Iv mg sulphate bolus **Dose :** 40mg/kg =,08ml/kg of mg sulphate 50% over 20 minute	

High Dependency Unit

1. Oxygen monitoring .
2. Fluid maintainance (2/3) maintainance   and open ryle
3. Continous salbutamol neublizer
4. Iv steriod /6hours
5. Mg sulphate bolus (if not given)
6. Iv salbutamol bolus
7. If no response after 20 minutes
   Start salbutamol or aminophylline infusion (two with other incompatabile)

Notes for exams

- Steriod effective only after 4-6 hours
- Iv steriods only if vomiting ,otherwise oral steriods.
- Spacers for all children even adults ,better deposition of inhaled medications
- Drip and dry method for spacer cleaning
- Steriods still of vital role in bronchial asthma exacerbation
- Benefits of steriod outweight its side effects
- Discharge patient from hospital if stable on 3-4 hourly B2 agonists .
- Pectus carinatum is sign of chronic asthma and not related to severity of asthma .
- Expected PEFR (L/M)=(height in cm – 80) x5 **important**
- (**Fop**)major factor for persistent asthma is atopic dermatitis and parent asthma .

Asthma Prophylaxis (Preventive Measures)

Step1	Step2	Step 3	Step4	Step5
Short acting B2 agonist as needed, to relieve manifestations indicated for all patients	>5 years low dose inhaled ICS=100-200 ug beclomethazone And Prn SABA	>5year -LTRA +low dose ICS **If not improved** -stop LTRA -start LABA+ low dose ICS **If not improved** -change to MART regimen with low ICS **If not improved :** -moderate dose inhaled cs= 200-4oo Either with -MART or -LABA And SABA As needed	>5 years -add slow release theophylline or -further increase dose ics =400- 800	>5 years -Exrecise challenge with spirometry to confirm diagnosis Then add regular oral corticosterio ds

	<5 years :	If < 5years :	<5 Years :	
	-8 weeks trial moderate dose ics =200-400 **If not improved** -consider other diagnosis **If improved** -stop for 8 weeks -if symptoms recurring within 4 weeks then start ICS in low dose as first line maintanance -if symptoms recurring beyond 4 weeks ,repeat 8 weeks another trial of moderate ICS	-Add LTRA -No increase dose of steriod	-Stop LTRA and Refere	

Methods of delivery : Spacer with mask -In mild to moderate exacerbation **Neublizer** -in severe exacerbation **dry powder inhaler** in >5 years age	Side effect low dose ICS -oral candidiasis -dysphonia So -mouth rinsing after use -use space		Side effect of high dose ICS -adrenal suppression -cataract -growth failure -purpura	

- **MART** :maintainance and reliever therapy =fast acting LABA
- **Aim is** :to achieve Best control at lowest dose .
- Gradual increase dose of steriod give better results than steady dose
- **When to stop ICS** : if on low dose ICS and symptomatic free
- Step down treatment if asthma controlled at least 3 months .
- If home neublizer not effective ,hospital admission is required

Uncontrolled asthma (guidelines)

>= 3 days /weeks with symtoms
>= days /weeks required use of SABA for symotomatic relief
>= one night /week awakening due to asthma

- Review response to treatment in 4-8 weeks
- Precaution before going to next step in uncontrolled asthma :
  - ✓ Check inhaler technique
  - ✓ Check for non compliance .
  - ✓ On going trigger factors .
  - ✓ Other diagnosis
  - ✓ Concomittant diseases

Diagnosis &Investigation Of Bronchial Asthma

- **<5 years with suspected asthma :**
  - o Diagnosis by clinical trial and observation .
- **>5 years :**
  - o Diagnosis by clinical and observation .
  - o if still symptoms do **objective tests** ,as shown in the following figure

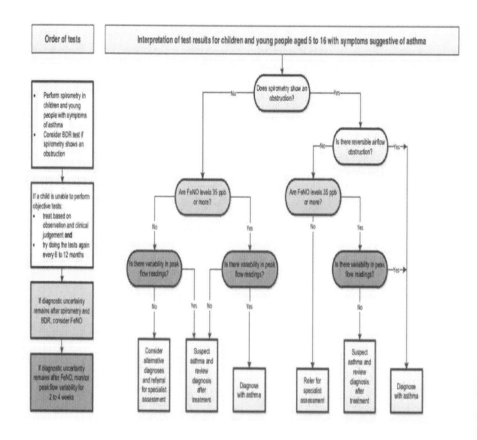

- **Chest xray for child with asthma exacerbation showing bilateral hyperexpansion and flat diaphragm** (Normal chest xray not rule out asthma)

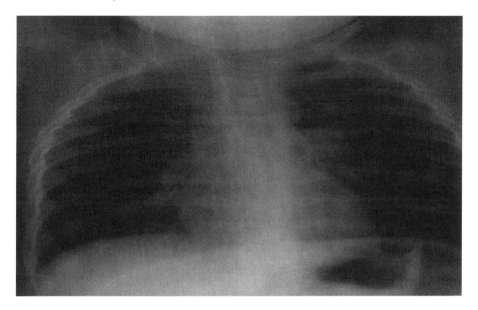

Chest xray for child with asthma presented with stabbing chest pain diagnosed as pneumomedistinum

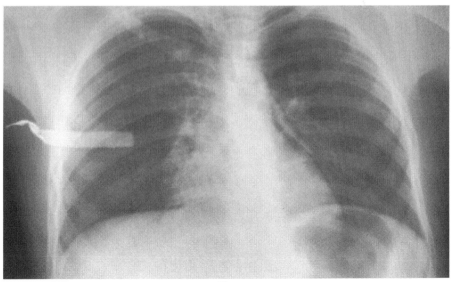

- Absence of bronchodilator reversibility not rule out asthma diagnosis
- Spirometry is done 15-20 minutes after giving brochodilator.

FEV1	PEFR
<ul><li>Forced expiratory volume of expired air in the first second after forced inspiration .</li><li>Only available with spirometry</li><li>Effort independent</li><li>Reflect moderate or large airways obstruction</li><li>Used in stable patients .</li><li>Gold standard for diagnosis of bronchial asthma : obstructive spirometry and positive bronchodilator reversibilty spirometry.</li></ul>	<ul><li>Easy</li><li>Single patient use</li><li>Clean once /wk</li><li>At home</li><li>Most useful</li><li>Effort dependent</li><li>Reflect large airway obstruction</li><li>Used After 6 years old age</li><li>Not substitutive for spirometry</li></ul> **Used** <ul><li>Assessment of asthma exacerbation</li><li>Diagnosis of bronchial asthma byserial PEFR</li></ul>
Interpretation :	
<ul><li>Fvc near normal >80% + low FEV1</li><li>Or FEV1: FVC <70% of predicted</li></ul> **DD** <ul><li>○ Restrictive as scoliosis</li><li>○ Mixed as cystic fibrosis</li></ul>	Variability >20% more than 3 days /week for 2-4 weeks = diagnose bronchial asthma

Complications Of Bronchial Asthma

- **Tension Pneumothorax**

    o Unilateral hyperresonance
    o Unilateral decrease air entry
    o If large or tension : chest tube
- **Pneumomediastinum (akp xray)**
    o Stabbing chest pain ,radiated to neck
    o Most common cause of pneumomediastinum is bronchial asthma

- **Respiratory failure rare**

Differential Diagnosis Of Wheezy Chest

1) **Acute**
   - Acute bronchiolitis
   - Bronchopneumonia
   - First episode of asthma
   - Forign body inhalation
   - Congestive heart failure

2) **Chronic**
   - Aspiration :
     o Gerd
     o Tracheoosophageal fistula (h type)
     o Forign body
   - Chronic infection:
     o Cystic fibrosis
     o Bronchiectasis
     o TB
     o PCD
     o Mycoplasma
     o Aggammaglobinemia

   - Extrinsic compression :
     o Vascular ring
     o Mediastinal syndrome

   - Brochiolitis obliterans
   - Tracheomalacia
   - Vocal cord dysfunction :
     o Vocal cord partially closed during inspiration
     o Cause exercise induced dyspnea
     o Poor response to beta 2 agonists
     o Cough
     o Shortness of breath
     o Chest and throat tightness
     o May be associated with asthma
     o Normal pefr
     o Diagnosis by flexible laryngeoscopy showing paradoxical movements of vocal cords
     o Refere to speech therapy to learn techniques for breathing control (akp)

Past Exams Questions For Bronchial Asthma

1. 11 years old boy who has asthma exacerbation , his PEFR is 150 l/min, the best recommendation is : go to emergency department
   Explanation : low PEFR indicating severe asthma
   Normal PEFR for this age is nearly 450l/minutes .

2. 12 years old boy with oxygen saturation 86%,unable to provide peak flow ,the best management : iv salbutamol
   Explanation : life threatening asthma

3. 6 years old girl known to be asthmatic ,unable to speak ,RR 50 /min,silent chest ,the best management : neublized salbutamol
   Explanation : severe asthma

4. 8 years old asthmatic boy with oxygen saturation 93% in air ,pefr 70% and rr=23 per minute ,the best management : salbutamol inhaler via spacer
   Explanation : mild to moderate exacerbation

5. Best diagnosis to exercise induced asthma : serial PEFR and normal base line spirometry
6. 2 month age baby with history of prematurity and intubation, come with wheezy chest,   diagnosis is : tracheomalacia
   Explanation : intubation is arisk factor for tracheomalacia

7. Chronic Dry cough only during day ,absent at night
   Diagnosis : habitual cough
   Explanation : asthma cough at night and early morning

2- BRONCHIOLITIS

- Acute viral infection of terminal bronchioles.
- RSV (it is most common cause of pneumonia in first 6 month of life)
- Highly contagious .
- spread by droplet .
- Hand washing is most effective way to prevent it .
- Occur in Winter and early spring .
- History of prematurity or mechanical ventilator is arisk factor .

Clinical Picture :

Prodroma of coryza last 1-3 days Followed by
- Difficult feeding
- Persistant cough
- Tachypnea and or chest recession
- Bilateral wheeze and crackles on auscultaion
  - wheeze commonly present but not essential for diagnosis
  - crackles often present =key finding
- Apnea especially if <6 weeks of age.
- Recurrent wheeze after bronchiolitis .

Indication Of Hospital Admission :

- RR > 60
- Difficult feeding or inadequate oral fluid intake
- Risk factors
- Clinical dehydration

Indication Of ICU Admission :

- Apnea observed or reported
- Severe RD
  - RR >70
  - Marked recession
  - Grunting
  - Central cyanosis
  - Persistant oxygen saturation in room air <92%

Risk Factor For Bronchiolitis :

- Maternaal smoking
- Low socioeconomic status
- Premature <32 weeks
- Male
- Not being Breast fed .

Risk Factor For Severe Bronchiolitis :

- Preexisting (BPD,CF)
- Congenital heart disease sor heart failure
- Hospitalized infant

Differential Diagnosis

- Lobar pneumonia
- Bronchopneumonia
- Viral induced wheeze
- Aspiration pneumonia
- Tracheomalacia
- Interstial pneumonitis
- GORD
- Congestive heart failure as vsd , svt,Tapvc, ALCAPA , myocarditis

Investigation

No routine investigation (fop) as the diagnosis is clinical .

- **Chest Xray :**

Indication :

1) Suspecting pneumonia (high fever ,focal crackles)
2) Prolonged illness.

Findings :

- o 30% atelectasis (right upper lobe or patchy)
- o Bilateral hyperinflation
- o Flat diaphragm .

- **Serum sodium done only if iv fluid is indicated**

- **PCR for RSV on nasopharyngeal aspirate : not routine**

<u>Complications Of Bronchiolitis :</u>

Bronchiolotis Obliterans :(AKP)

- Adenovirus
- Age 16-20 month
- Also brochiolitis obliterans may follow graft transplantation
- Granulation tissues in bronchioles lumen
- Previously well
- Acute brochiolits , with extended course over weeks without improvement
- chest deformity

Clinical picture

- No clinical signs of infections
- Fatigue ,weight loss **=charactarestic**
- **Triade :**
  1) Chronic dry cough
  2) Chronic or persistant RD on exertion
  3) Chronic wheeze , not responding to Bronchodilator or inhaled steroids

Examination:

- Crepitations
- Clubbing

Investigation :

- Chest Xray:
  - o Unilateral hemitranslucent chest
- Ct chest
- Lung function tests
- Biobsy: confirm dx

Treatment :

- Antibiotics of no benefits
- Trial of inhaled steroids to rule out asthma

Treatment Of Bronchiolitis

Nice Guidline advise us not to use routinely the following drugs :

- Antibiotics
- Hypertonic saline
- Neublized adrenaline
- Neublized salbutamol
- Montelokast
- Ipratropium bromide
- Systemic or inhaled corticosteroids

Main Treatment :   **Supportive Treatment (AKP)**

1) Humidified o2 if saturation <92%
2) Suction
3) Hydration
   So only **cardio respiratory monitoring** for apnea detection

1. **Humidified warmed O2**   ⟶   **CPAPA ....MV**
   - Via head box or nasal prong
   - Not use mask
   - Nasal prong Not effective if
     - Baby is mouth breather
     - Blocked nose

2. **Suction :**
   Not routine

Indication

- RD
- Feeding difficulties because of airway obstruction
- Apnea even if no obvious upper airway secretion(reported apnea)
- Noisy breathing or nasal congestion

3. Hydration

- Oral or NGT or iv only if not tolerate oral or NGT
- 7o ml/kg/day
- D5% ,9 NaCl
- Follow up serum NA
- Change to ,45%NaCl

Palvizumab :

Indication Of Vaccine Palivizumab:

- Born< 35wks + <= 6 month at the start of RSV season
- <2 years old +received treatment for BPD within last 6 month
- <2 years old+ significant Congenital heart disease

Given IM ,Monthly

Ribavarin

- Difficult administration(inhaler for 12-20 hours per day for 5 days
- Very expensive
- Not drug of choice as limited effectiveness against RSV.
- Given if risk of severe bronchiolitis
- Teratogenic

Past Exams Question For Bronchiolitis

1. 6 month old infant with wide spread wheeze and crepitation ,his saturation is 89%,best management is to give only oxygen without salbutamol

    Explanation : a case of bronchiolitis(not bronchial asthma),no place for salbutamol

2. 6 month old infant with wide spread wheeze and crepitation ,his saturation is 89%, gallop and hepatomegally , best management is surgical treatment

    Explanation a case of TAPVC supracardiac type

    Remember that no viral prodroma in congestive heart failure

3. 6 weeks old girl with cough and dyspnea .chest xray shows hyperinflation and interstial infilterate ,was treated with chloramphenicol eye drops for conjunctivitis ,diagnosis is Chlamydia pneumonia

    Explanation history of conjunctivitis is clue for Chlamydia pneumonia

4. 4 month infant with fever,cough ,reduced feeding ,RR 60/minutes

    Diagnosis is bronchiolitis

3- PNEUMONIA

Etiology :

Community Acquired Pneumonia :

- **Viral**
    - o RSV :Most common cause of CAP <6 month
    - o most common in younger children
    - o 35 % of childhood pneumonia
- **Bacterial**
    - o Sterptococcus pneumonia>6 month
    - o Mycoplasma >5 years
    - o Chlamydia
    - o Klibsiella

Hospital Acquired Pneumonia :

- Associated with Mechanical Ventilation .
- Intrinsic neurological or respiratory abnormalities
    - o Gram negative pneumonia
    - o Staph aureus
    - o Fungel infection
    - o Hemophilus influenza
    - o Liogonella ,pcp,lymphocytic interstitial pneumonia

Pathological Classification :

- **Lobar pneumonia (typical)**
    streptococcus pneumonia
- **Bronchopneumonia (atypical and viral)**

Clinical picture :

- **Lobar pneumonia (Typical pneumonia) :**
    -It is Difficult to locate focal signs (crackles) in the first six month

-If <3 years old , lobar pneumonia considered if :

- Fever >38.5
- Chest recession
- Respiratory distress > 50/minute
  Often the only clue to diagnosis is tachypnea .

  - **Chest Examination :**
    - o   Bronchial breathing
    - o   Consonating crepitation
    - o   Dullness on percussion
    - o   Decrease air entry
  - **Indication criteria of admission :**
    - o   History of apnea or cyanosis
    - o   Age < three month
    - o   Impaired immune function
    - o   Poor social situation of follow up
    - o   Pleural Effusion
    - o   Not tolerate oral or dehydrated or toxic appearance

Investigation :

- Measure O2 saturation
- CBC-CRP
  - o   add nothing to treatment
  - o   Not differentiate viral from bacterial
  - o   Only for follow up
- Blood cultures : performed for all pneumonic patients needing hospitilizations.
- Sputum culture : difficult to obtained in children
- Chest xray :
  - o   not routine in mild uncomplicated lower respiratory tract infection
  - o   Indicated for hospitalized cases or un certain diagnosis or suspected complication
  - o   Indication to repeat xray :
    - ☒   Round pneumonia
    - ☒   Lobar collapse
    - ☒   Pleural effusion
    - ☒   Non resolved symptoms

Treatment

- All with clear diagnosis of pneumonia ,antibiotics whether bacteria or viral
- If abscent admission criteria :
  - First line antibiotic is **oral amoxicillin for one week**(fop)
    As it is effective against the majority of pathogens
  - Add macrolides at any age :
    - o if no response to the first line
    - o very severe disease
    - o if 5 years or older = first line is macrolides
  - Oral antibiotics are safe and effective even in severe Community acquired pneumonia .
- Iv antibiotics : only if not tolerate oral
- Physiotherapy : not benefiscial

Common Pneumonias

Strept Pneumonia	Staph Aureus	Klibsiella
->6 month -The most common pneumonia	Risk factors : -hospitalized or immunocompromized - staph skin infection -<1 year	=bronchiectasis sicca hemorragicca=as it colonizes upper airway
Clinical Picture		
-Focal crackles -No wheeze -Fever -RD -Chest pain -Round pneumonia -Pleural effusion is common (parapneumonic effusion) **Clinical picture :** o Original chest infection improve but after days ,fever develop again with progressive SOB o Dry cough o Progressive RD o Unilateral decrease Air entry o Unilateral dullness o Blood culture	-Very high fever -Pneumatocele o Constant feature o Multiple Air filled or fluid filled o May rupture causing pneumothorax, ,quickly lethal if no rapid treatment -Empyema and pyopneumothorax o clinical picture rather than complication= deteriorating despite antibiotics o air fluid level o mediastinal shift in	-Lobar pneumonia -Sputum culture = muciod colonies -Hemorragic pleural effusion =right upper lobe -Pneumatocele -Abcess

and iv antibiotics ○ Initial chest xray ○ Confirm with **chest us** To differentiate loculated (require surgical treatment) from non loculated ○ Chest drain insertion pig tail catheter (**small**) preferred than large bore(**akp**)	chest xray ○ need urgent iv **cefuraxime** ○ chest ultrasound and then chest drainage under anaesthesia (no thoracocentesis or ct chest)(**AKP**)	
Chest Xray		
(not indicated in uncomplicated CAP) **(fop)**	-Bilateral cavitating -bronchopneumonia	
Treatment :		
Oral Amoxicillin 7 days	Iv vancomycin	3rd generation cephalosporins

Mycoplasma	Pneumocystitis carnii	Chlamydia
-Preschool age -Referred as walking pneumonia As hospitalization is rare -it is bacteria but with no cell wall	**Risk factors :** -Immunocompromized : -HIV =40% of children with AIDs =afrocaribbian -Malignant disease on chemotherapy **Onset :** -In first year (mainly <4 year s old age) - high mortality	-common cause of pneumonia less than four months age
Clinical picture		
(gradual onset) -Low grade fever -Headache -Dry spasmodic chronic cough then become productive -Pharyngitis -Erythema multiform **(AKP)**	-Dry cough ,severe RD . -Desaturation =hypoxia is cardinal feature . -Rare extrapulmonary manifestations .	-Genetically infected mother -Afebrile 100% -History of conjunctivitis in 50% of cases -Staccatto cough -Tachypnea

Others : -Hepatitis -Autimmune hemolytic anemia (**AKP**) -Arthiritis -Encephalitis ,GBS -Myocarditis -Pleuritic chest pain **Signs : mild** Wheeze ,crepitatation	**Signs : mild** Wheeze ,crepitation	**Signs :mild** crackles ,wheeze
Investigations		
Chest xray : -Worse than symptoms and signs -Bilateral patchy consildation=butterfly -Small pleural effusion -Hilar LN **Laboratory :** **CBC . (AKP)** to exclude hemolytic anemia	**Chest xray :** -Bilateral infilterate =granular or butterfly **The best for diagnosis :** -Bronchoscopy with bronchoalveolar lavage -Lymphopenia -Incease LDH in 90% of patiants -No serology	**Chest Xray :** -Bilateral hyperexpansion -Symmetrical interstial infilterate

PCR for nasal washing = best test to confirm diagnosis **Gram stain .** -Polymorph without any bacteria **Culture difficult .** **Cold agglutinin .** -previously used -rising mycoplasma igM titre.		
Treatment		
-oral Macrolides -Lack of response to penicillin -BD and physiotherapy -antibiotics Not change course of disease	-High dose Sulfa methoxazole /TMP -Intravenous hydrocortisone **-if not improved** give pentamide iv or neublized **Prophylaxis :** -Sulpha /TMP -Dapsone	-oral Macrolides Clear conjunctivitis Prevent pneumonia later - Topical treatment of conjunctivitis Not prevent pneumonia later

Chest Xray   of **PCP** pneumonia of infant 2 months old age with **HIV**

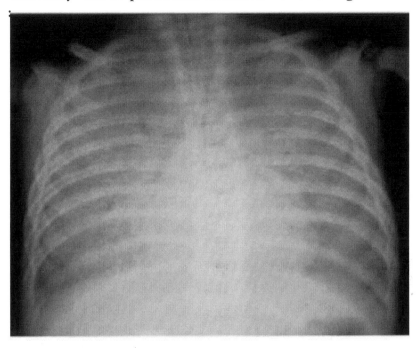

Chest Xray for infant 2 years old with round pneumonia :

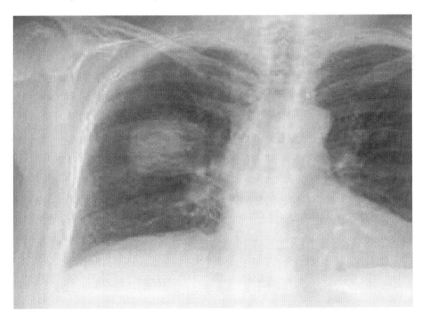

Chest Xray for child 4 years old with Mycoplasma Pneumonia :

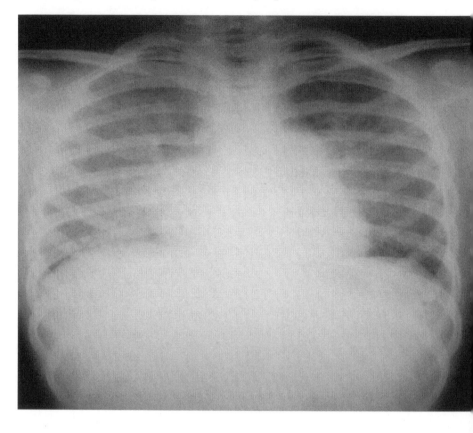

Past Exams Questions For Pneumonia

1. Pleural effeusion management : small pore chest drain
   Explanation :small pore chest drain comfortable than wide pore chest drain in effusion
2. HIV infant with hypoxemia and cough
   Diagnosis : PCP
   Explanation : clue is hypoxemia and immunocompromized infant
3. 5 years old boy with symmetrical rash on extremities and chronic cough
   Diagnosis : mycoplasma
   Explanation : Erythema multiform in preschool child with chronic cough is mycoplasma
4. Infant with high fever ,focal crackles ,diagnosis is streptococcus pneumonia
5. Chest Xray of round pneumonia **(AKP)**
6. Chest Xray for mycoplasma **(AKP)**

4- CYSTIC FIBROSIS

- AR
- Multisystem disease
- Most common Life threatening genetic disorder in Caucasian .
- Neonatal screening at Day five of age
    - Prevent early nutritional defeciencies
    - Improve long term growth
- Chronic infection limited to airways (airways disease)
- Severity varies among siblings
- Abnormal gene (cf transmembrane receptors) (CFTR)on long arm of chromosome 7
    - Decrease cl secretion(blocked channel)
    - Increase absorption of sodium
- salty taste, salt frosting of the skin
- Mixed lung disease (obstructive early then restrictive)
- Mutation :
  Most common mutation is delta phenyalanine 508 in 70%

    - Strongly associated with pancreatic insufficiency
    - More severe symptoms

Clinical Picture

Respiratory

(in 95%of patient)

Upper :

- Nasal polyps (cystic fibrosis is most common cause of nasal polyps ,and should be excluded in any case of nasal polyps especially if associated with growth failure)

Lower :

- Difficult asthma
    - Productive cough
    - RD
    - Recurrent wheeze

- Allergic bronchopulmonary aspergillosis
    - o Occur in cystic fibrosis and asthma (allergic reaction)
    - **Clinical picture :**
    - o Recurrent wheeze
    - o Dry cough
    - o Brownish plug in sputum (rusty)
    - o Central bronchiectasis
    - o No response to antibiotics
    - **Chest Xray:**
    - o Patchy round apical infilterate
    - o Transient
    - o Recurrent
    - o At different sites
    - **Diagnosis :**
    - o Peripheral osinophilia
    - o Total igE >1000
        - **Confirm by :**
    - o Positive aspergilous antigen skin test
    - o   Aspergilous IgE antibody
    - **Treatment :**

    - o oral prednisone 6 months
    - o antifungal drugs

- bronchiolitis :
    - o If with growth failure exclude cystic fibrosis

- Bronchiectasis
    - o Irreversible dilatation of bronchial tree
    - o Chronic ,persistant cough
    - o Productive of greenish ,copieus sputum
    - o Clubbing
    - o Course crepitation
    - o Other common causes of bronchiectasis :
        - ▪ Pertussis
        - ▪ Primary ciliary dyskinesia
        - ▪ Immunodeficiency
        - **Diagnosis**
    - o **Initial xray** : linear atelectasis peribronchial
    - o high resolution CT confirm diagnosis

- Recurrent Pneumonia

  - o Increase respiratory symptoms means infective exacerbation till proved otherwise
    - o Measure o2 saturation
    - o Do chest xray for focal changes and to follow response to treatment
    - o sputum culture
    - o lung function
  - o **Organisms :**

<2 years :
- o Staph
- o Non capsular hemophilus

>2 years :

- o Pseudomonas aurginosa
- o Stenotrophomonas maltophilia
- o Atypical mycobacterium
- o Burkholderia cepacia complex ,highly transmitted by epidemics .

Complication of cystic fibrosis :

- Hemoptysis (common)
- Core pulmonale (late)
- Pneumothorax & atelectasis in adults and adolescence
- Respiratory failure

GIT

- Delayed passage of meconium
- Meconium ileus in NB
- Ileal obstruction with fecal matter = meconium ileus equivalent in older children(distal intestinal obstruction syndrome)**AKP**
  - o Acute onset periumbilcal pain (right lower quadrant)
  - o Abdominal Mass
  - o Bilious vomiting abdominal distension
  - **Abdominal Xray**
  -Air fluid level if negative do abdominal us or ct

Treatment :
- o Hydration
- o Gastrographi oral or enteral (first line treatment)
- o Oral Macrogel
- Constipation
- Piles
- Intussucception especially in older than one year (AKP)
- Rectal prolapse in 10%
- GERD

Pancreas

(**85% of patient**)
- ✓ FTT begin in first few months of life
- ✓ Malabsorption of fat and protein .
- ✓ Steatorrhea & fat soluble vitamins deficiency (rickets , ataxia , bleeding tendency)
- ✓ foul smelling ,pale ,bulky , greasy stool .
- ✓ Hypoproteinemia and edema
- ✓ DM develop later on after 10 years in 5-8%
  - 25% at 20 years
  - 75% at 30 years
  - 5% eventually develop DM, Annaualy from 10 years
  - DM diagnosis is **Suspected If**
    - o Preceeded by deteriorating lung function
    - o Increase frequency of chest exacerbation
    - o Unexplained wt loss
  - Often straightforward to control
  - Of adult type
  - Ketoacidosis uncommon
  - **Diagnosis of choice** : oral glucose tolerance not fasting
  - If abnormal OGT test perform continuous glucose monitoring to confirm diagnosis
  - Treatment : **diet and insulin** if no response to diet control (no oral hypoglycemic)

Hepatic

- Neonatal hepatitis , conjugated hyperbilirubinemia (prolonged NB jaundice)
- Hepatomegally.**(not in celiac disease)**
- Cirrhosis is very late sign ,occur in adults.
- Hepatic cirrhosis uncommon but can occur in children .
- Liver cell failure ,Portal hypertension due to focal biliary cirrhosis in in 25% .

Urogenital

- Males
  - Azospermia
  - 99% will be infertile
- Female
  - Cervicitis
  - Abnormal thick cervical secretion
  - Many girls infertile .

Sweat

- Hypokalemia
- Metabolic alkalosis
- Hyponatremia
- Hypocholermia
 (Pseudobartter)

Diagnosis :

One of clinical presentation   +   one of CFTR dysfuntion

• Positive Newborn screening • Sibling diagnosed cystic fibrosis • At least one clinical signs	• Two positive sweat chloride tests • 2 CF mutations • Abnormal NPD

Common exams Scenarios For AKP And FOP :

A. Newborn +prolonged jaundice +delayed passage of meconium >36 hours +FTT
B. Growth failure +constipation +recurrent wheeze + productive cough
C. Growth failure +recurrent wheeze +pneumonia +lab of pseudobartter
D. Short stature +delayed puberty+nasal polyp
E. DM child +growth failure +respiratory problems
F. Growth failure +clubbing + low serum sodium
G. Growth failure +recurrent chest infection +persistant nasal discharge > 6 month
H. Hepatomegally and malabsorption not celiac disease but cystic fibrosis

Investigation :

Sweat cl test	Indication : • Any unexplained respiratory symptoms • Or git symptoms • Still gold standard for diagnosis • Still most reliable test • New method macroduct <100 mg sweat • Skin burn if unbuffered solution used **False positive :** • Adrenal insufficiency • Hypothyroidism • Hypopituatarism • Hypoparathyriodism • Pseudohypoaldostertonism • Nephrotic syndrome • Nephrogenic DI • Ectodermal dysplasia • Eczyma **False negative :** • Hypopntemia ,edema • Preterm • Less than two weeks age **Tests :** • Collect 100 mg of sweat • Only for 20-30 min • Measure cl

	Precautions : • Performed after 2-3 weeks age **Interpretation** • Cl tend to be > na • Cl > 60 very suggestive of CF • Na not interpreted in absence Of cl . • Sum of cl and Na >140

Respiratory function tests	• Low FVC
	• Much lower FEV1
	• Diff between FEV1 and FVC >25%
	• FEV1 :FVC <70
	• **FEV1**
	   ○ <30%= very poor prognostic sign
	   ○ It measure lung function in cf
	   ○ Indicate prognosis when measured over time
	
	Lung clearance index done if normal spirometry

Radiological	• Hyperexpansion of lung • Flat diaphragm • Bronchiectasis (peribronchial thickening)

Pancreatic functions	• Low stool elastase
	• High immunoreactive trypsinogen
	   (best screening test)
	   If positive do genetic test on same sample
	• Increase fecal fat
	• Pancreatic function worsen over time

Bacteriological	• Sputum culture
Gene analysis	• Definitive diagnosis • Negative genotype not exclude diagnosis • Antenatal diagnosis only if obligate carrier with one child cystic fibrosis

Treatment

Admission only in severe cases

Pulmonary therapy	A. **Sputum Staph**
	-Flucloxacillin prophylacis from diagnosis till 3 yrs
	-If positive culture while on prophylaxis ,review adherence ,treat by antistaph antibiotics
	
	Pseudomonas
	  i. **Symptomatic clinical unwell**
	
	    Antibiotics :
	    -ivCeftazidime
	    -inhaled Tobramycin
	    Dose: 2-3 times dt high clearance of abs
	
	  ii. **Clinically well**
	    Start three weeks of :
	
	    -Oral cipromycin
	    -Neublized colomycin **(if not tolerated ..neublized tobramycin**
	
	B. **Neublized antibiotics**
	C. **Oral antibiotics**
	  • Only on discharge
	D. **Bronchodilator s :**
	  • Salbutamol MDI+spacer
	  • Before chest physiotherapy
	E. **Inhaled corticosteroids**
	  No evidence benefits

Nutrition	• Affect life expectancy • High calories diets o No fat restriction • Vitamins and minerals(ADEK)

	• Pancreatic enzyme replacement
	   ○ Before all meals and snacks
	   ○ Fibrosing clonopathy (side effects of pancreatic enzymes)
	• Salt supplement
	   ○ Not routine
	   ○ Only in summer

Recent advances	**Pulmozyme** Single daily arosol • Improve pulmonary function • Hydrolyze Dna in mucous • Decrease viscosity
Physiotherapy	• Twice daily • Prevent and treatmeny of chest infection • Exercise encouraged but not substitute for physiotherapy
Surgery	Lung and heart transplantation IF irreversible respiratory failure
Immunoregulatory	If cystic fibrosis +deteriorating lung function or repeated exacerbation Azithromycin used long term In no effect give oral corticosteroid (not inhaled)
Prognosis :	65% diagnosed in first year 10% not diagnosed till 10 years Life expectancy 40 yr

5- STRIDOR

- Clinical diagnosis
- Imaging not routine for diagnosis
- noisy breathing
- Inspiratory stridor (laryngeal obstruction)
- Expiratory stridor (obstructed lower trachea)
- Biphasic = glottic or subglottic causes

Mild =grade 1	Moderate =grade 2	Severe =grade 3 ,4
First line :	First line :	-O2 face mask if saturation <92% -Neublized adrenaline used only in severe cases to buy time for intubation
Dexamethazone	Dexamethazone	(Only transient effect)
- 150micro g/kg - Oral advantage : less distress - IM if unable to swallow	- 150micro g/kg - Oral	-call anaesthetic for ETT
Budeosonide	Budeosonide	If failed intubation: Tracheostomy (ENT)
- 2mg - Neublized	- 2mg - Neublized	
		- Iv antibiotics **so,** late cannulation **Cefotaxime** is the antibiotic of choice in

		acute epiglottitis
o Both equally effective o More effective than prednisolone o Onset of action after 90 minutes		
Home treatment : -Mists tents (humidified air) **not** proven to be beneficial	-Observe for 4 hours for RD or increasing stridor **If worsening :** -Neublized adrenaline 5ml of 1:1000 And further observation	-Head tilt and chin lift -Avoid distressing child during examination (risk of complete airway obstruction) -Throat should not be examined **Causes of severe stridor:** -Epigllotitis -Trachetitis -FB inhalation
-Exertion stridor =only on crying	-Stridor at rest =continous	-Stridor with retraction -Stridor with cyanosis

Acute Stridor

1. Infectious

Acute spasmodic laryngitis	Acute Laryngiotrache obronchitis	Acute Tracheitis	Acute epiglottits
	-Most coomon -Clinical diagnosis	May sequale of Laryngeotracheo bronchitis	-Medical emergency -Age (6month-6 years)
Etiology			
-No prodroma -Upper airway reactivity - personal Atopy -Positive FH of atopy - Recurrence is common	-Viral infection of Vocal C ord -Parainfluenza -6 months - 4 years	-Bacterial infection of trachea and larynx -Staph or strept pneumonia	**-H influenza** -Contagious -Rare cause -Decrease incidence with HIB vaccine but not eliminate it -So History of missed vaccination will suspect the diagnosis
Clinical picture			
-Recurrent Croup>=2 per year	-Mild fever coryza		**-no history of upper respiratory tract**

			infection
-Stridor	-Well appearance		
		-Gradual onset	-Short history
- may Require investigations to exclude anatomical airway abnormalities by direct laryngscopy or bronchoscopy	-Barking cough		-Sudden onset over hours
	-Biphasic stridor = characterstics		-High fever>38
		-High fever	
	-Hoarseness ,aphonia are common	-No 3D	-dyspnea , dysphonia
			,dysphagia
	-May be RD grade 1 or 2	-Cough	-No cough
		-No drooling	-Drooling and neck extension
			-Tripod position
Investigation			
	Xray neck AP -Steeple sign= narrowing of subglottic space		**Lateral neck xray** -Positive thumb print once airway secured
		Laryngeoscopy: Pseudomembrane	**Laryngeoscopy:** Large edematous cherry red epiglottis
Treatment			
- Steroids not	-Self limiting	**As severe**	**As severe**

indicated	-Racemic epinephrine not first line **-Oral or inhaled steroids**	**stridor**	**stridor**

2. Non infectious

Forign Body inhalation	Laryngeal spasm	Laryngeal edema (angioneurotic edema)anaphyl actic shock	Laryngeal compression (retropharynge al abcess)
-Toddler 6m-5yr -Commonly right main bronchus As it is More vertical	-Vitamin D deficiency -Autoimmune hypoparathyriodism (Digorge)	See gatroentrology	-Primary infection in head and neck (Complication of bacterial pharyngitis) which inturn drain retropharyngeal lymph nodes -Group ABH strept.
Clinical picture -Sudden onset in previously well child + failure to respond to neublized salbutamol -Unilateral Decrease AE - localized			**Clinical picture** -High fever -Dysphagia -Drooling -Distress -Neck hyperextension

wheeze -Subsequent Pneumonia -History of chocking -Abrupt cough -Recurrent pneumonia in the same area			**Examination :** -Cervical LN -Flactaunt mass
-Lateral Decubitus xray: **Or** **inspiratory and expiratory film** if co operative **-chest us or flurouscopy** **-Bronchoscopy Rigid :** Diagnostic and therapeutic **Chest xray or us done prior to it .** **Treatment :** -See severe Stridor -Rigid bronchoscopy , Antibiotics -If persistent signs after initial			**-Lateral neck xray :** -Increase retropharyngeal or prevertebral Soft tissue =bulge in post pharyngeal wall **Ultrasound of neck** Confirm diagnosis But most appropriate is **CT** **Treatment :** **If airway compromised :** Surgical incision and drainage **If airway not compromised :** Iv clindamycin

Bronchoscopy ,repeat bronchoscopy,do -venitilation /perfusion scan			

Lateral neck Xray for Child with epiglottitis

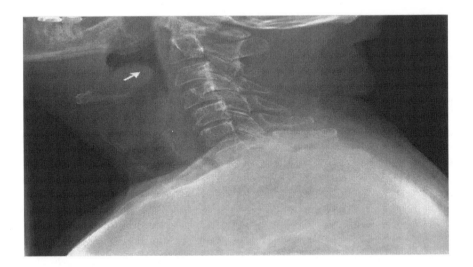

Lateral Xray neck for child with retropharyngeal abcess

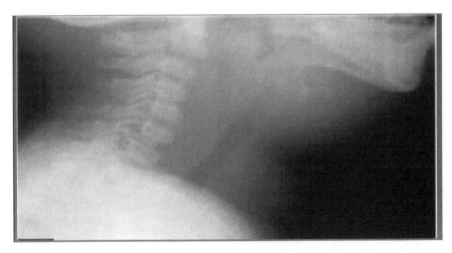

Chronic stridor
A. Congenital chronic stridor

Laryngeomalacia	Tracheomalacia	Choanal atresia	Laryngeal tumours =subglottic hemangioma	Laryngeal web
-Most common cause of persistant stidor in infancy 60-70% **Larynx** disproportionally small so ,collapse or narrowing during inspiration will occur.	**Causes :** -Idiopathic -BPD -Intubation -GERD	-It is the most common congenital anomaly of nose -May be associated with charge syndrome - Microphthalmia -Heart defect		Most at vocal cord
Onset : -At birth or NB	**Onset :** -Typically in 2nd month of life			
Clinical Picture				
-Thrive and feed normally **-Stridor :** -Inspiratory -Only noisy breathing -Increase by crying ,feeding .	-Exp wheeze Uniform in all lung field -Misdiagnosed as Bronchial asthma or CF or prolonged bronchiolitis But :	- Unsuccessful extubation -Cyanosis on feeding or suckling -relieved by crying -Difficult to pass catheter	Suspected if -neck hemangioma or naevus -Stridor increasing with time (**fop**	-Stridor from birth -Weak cry -Biphasic stridor =critical UAO -Recurrent croup in

		through each nostril 3-4 cm into nasopharynx	) -No RD	infancy
-Not heared at rest or sleep.	Bronchodilator worsen symptoms			
	- named Happy wheezer	-Difficult feeding , Chocking and cyanosis		
Investigations				
Bronchoscopy	Bronchoscopy	CT	MRI	
-Long ,folded, omega shaped epiglottis	-Most accurate -show Collapse on expiration	-After stabilization and maintainance of patent airway		
-For exclusion of laryngeal web or cysts	**Confirmed by :** Fluoroscopy of airway ....narrowing with expiration			
Indication : -Stridor at rest				
-Late presentation				
-FTT				
-Persistant or severe or - biphasic stridor				
Prognosis : -Resolve by 18 months	**Prognosis :** -Excellent resolve by 3 years			

Treatment				
-Self limited(reassurance) -Rarely ,3% tracheostomy when life threatening apnea or airway obstruction	-treatment of cause -Avoid BD -Systemic steroid in exacerbation - Tracheostomy Surgery if recurrent pneumonia or FTT ,vascular ring	-Initial : placement of **Oral airway** or oral airway intubation - Tracheostomy if patient has potentially life threating problems		

Congenital Laryngeal Compression

Causes

- **Vascular ring**
- **Congenital goiter**
- **Pierre robbin sequence**
- **Cystic hygroma**

Vascular   ring

≤6 months

- Feeding difficulities (apnea)
- Stridor
- Wheeze
    - Worse with time
    - Worse during feeding and neck flexion during sleep
    - Relieved by neck extension .

> 6 months

- Dysphagia
- Chocking   ,recurrent pneumonia.

Diagnosis :

-Gold standard (gastrographin swallow)

-neck MRI

Treatment : surgical repair   (life saving)

B. Acquired chronic stridor

Subglottic stenosis	Mediastinal syndrome	Bilateral vocal cord paralysis
-Not improve with time -Stridor not increasing -bi phasic ,static -No RD -History of intubation	-Worsening stridor -Wheeze on lying flat -Pale -Lethargic -Worsening noisy breathing -Cervical LN enlargement	-Shortly after birth -Moderate RD due progressive airway obstruction -Stable stridor inspiratory or biphasic -stridor at rest that worsen upon agitation -Weak cry or near normal

	Differential diagnosis	
	-Thymus where there is no compression of large airway and lung tissues visible through the structure . If any doubt do **chest ultrasound**	**If unilateral vocal cord paralysis :** -Weak cry or hoarse sound -Aspiration : Recurrent chocking and cough not related to food **Etiology :** -Ventouse delivery following failed forceps -Birth trauma -Open heart surgery -Cns anomalies as hydrocephalus

Acase of mediastinal widening diagnosed as lymphoma

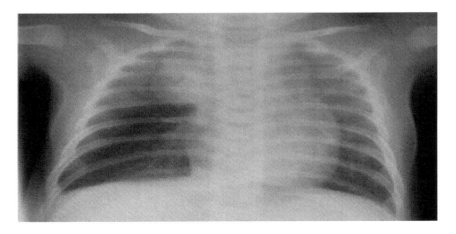

6 - PRIMARY CILIARY DYSKINESIA

Clinical Picture

In 50% of cases : Situs inversus + dextrocardia = kartagner syndrome

- **Triade Of Diagnosis :**

  - Cough (principle symptom),productive ,chronic or recurrent.
  - Chronic sinusitis =Runny nose from birth, frontal headache is clue for sinusitis .
  - Recurrent Otitis Media= Conductive Hearing loss, often treated

- **Late Finding :**

  - Recurrent pneumonia & bronchiectasis
  - recurrent wheeze = misdiagnosed as asthma
  - growth failure

Complication :

- Nasal polyp
- Clubbing
- Infertility

Investigations :

-Chest xray :

- Hyperexpansion
- Infilterate
- Dextrocardia in kartagner syndrome
- Bronchiectasis

-Screening test : Low exhaled nitric oxide = suggest diagnosis

-Respiratory function test : early obstructive, late mixed

-Microscopy of cilia for motility =confirm diagnosis

Treatment :

- Supportive
- BD
- Mucolytics
- Physiotherapy
- Immunization
- aggressive treatment of infection

Prognosis

- Normal life span
- Symptoms tend to improve after adolescence

Chest Xray for child with bronchiectasis :

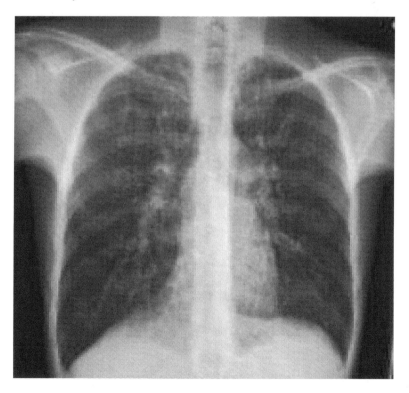

Chest Xray for newborn with kartagner syndrome :

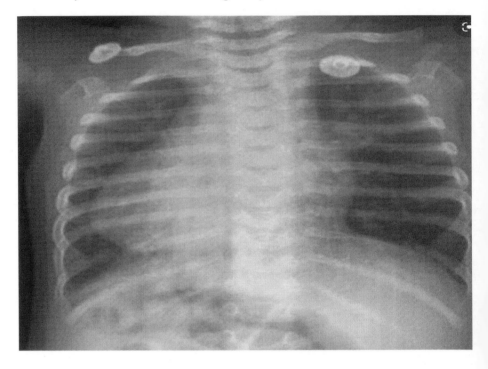

7- CONGENITAL LUNG MALFORMATION

Congenital lobar emphysema	Congenital cystic adenomatous malformation	Pulmonary sequestration	Bronchogenic cyst
-Most common **Onset :** -Newborn - at 2-6 month (more common) -More in male	-2nd most common **Onset :** Newborn	-Mass of non functioning pulmonary tissues -No bronchial communication	-Budding of trachea -Rarely present in newborn
Site			
-Left upper lobe is most common -rarely affect lower lobes	-right upper lobe	-Extra lobar in left lower lobe	-Right side near midline
Clinical Picture			
-May asymptomatic -Respiratory distress -Majority not diagnosed antenatal	-may be asymptomatic -RD -recurrent chest infection -may undiscovered for years ,present	-Recurrent unilateral pneumonia in left lower lobe (same area)	-Recurrent chest infection -DD round pneumonia

	later by spontaneous pneumothorax but persistant chest radiographic abnormalities after chest tube insertion		
Examination : -Unilateral -Decrease air entry over affected lobe -Shift of cardiac beat to opposite side **(DD dextrocardia)** -Assymmetry of chest			
Chest Xray			
-Hyperinflation of affected lobe (hypertranclucent hemithorax) -Compression of adjacent lung tissues -Herniation in superior mediastinum -Shift of medistinum to opposite side -Presence of BV marking within	-Normal appearance of gas in abdomen -Shift of mediastinum to contralateral side -Normal diaphragm contour -Multicystic **DD (Congenital diaphragmatic hernia)**	**Chest Xray review :** Important for diagnosis **Chest us :** Initial to exclude diaphragmatic hernia which present in 40-50% of cases	

emphesamtous lobe **Best to confirm diagnosis :** CT			
Treatment			
Asymptomatic -Conservative treatment only **Symptomatic** -lobectomy	-frequently surgical excision due to increase risk of neoplasm		-Surgical excision if symptomatic

Chest Xray for 2 month infant with congenital lobar emphysema :

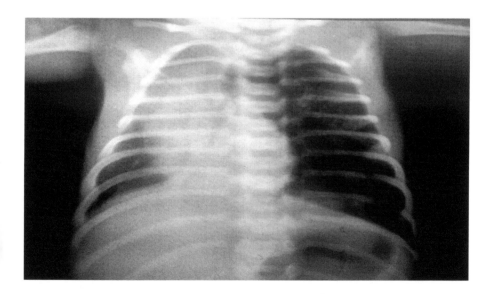

Chest xray of newborn with right congenital cystic adenomatous malformation

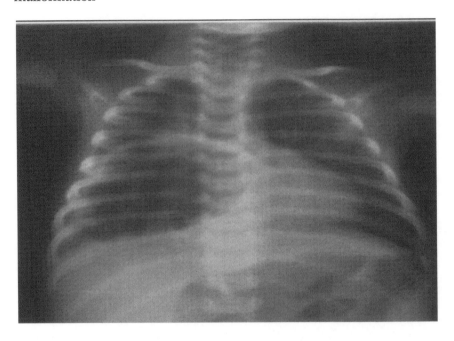

Chest Xray newborn with congenital diaphragmatic hernia :

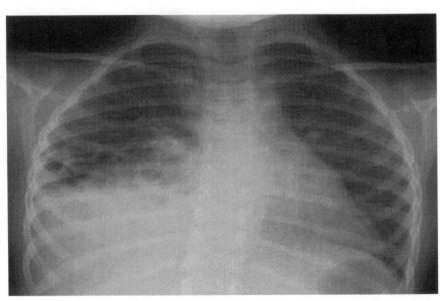

Eventration of diaphragm	Congenital diaphragmativ hernia
-Thin diaphragmatic muscle **Risk factor :** Obstructed labour	-Mainly on left side
Clinical Picture	
Onset : NB or during infancy -Asymptomatic -Severe RD on resuscitation -may be Erbs palsy also -Persistent or chronic cough	**Onset: NB or beyond neonatal period** -RD in first few hours after birth **Examination :** -Scaphiod abdomen -Displacement of heart beat to contralateral side
Investigations	
Initial Xray **Chest ultrasound :** Confirm diagnosis	**Initial Xray :** Usually diagnostic **Chest ultrasound :** Confirm diagnosis
Treatment	
-If asymptomatic : no treatment -If symptomatic : surgery	-Insert **large bore nasogastric tube** -Suction to prevent distension of intrathoracic bowel -Sedation ,paralysis and mechanical ventilation at low pip (gentle - ventilation)

8- INTERPRETATION OF SPIROMETRY

1. **Obstructive spirometry (bronchial asthma)**

   - Fvc near normal >80%
   - Low FEV1 <80%
   - FEV1 : FVC is low <70% of predicted

2. **Restrictive spirometry (scoliosis)**

   - FVC is low
   - FEV1 low
   - Difference between less than 2 5%
   - FEV1:FVC > 80%

3. **Mixed spirometry (cystic fibrosis)**

   - FVC low
   - FEV1 a lot lower
   - Difference between more than 25%
   - FEV1 :FVC is low < 70%

9- RESPIRATORY FAILURE

Respiratory Failure (Type 1)	Respiratory Failure (Type 2)	ARDS
-Hypoxic normocapnea or hypocapnea due to compensatory hyperventilation	-Hypoxic hypercapnea	-Non cardiogenic pulmonary edema -Resp failure type 1
Causes		
• Pneumonia • Pul embolism • Pul edema • ARDS • Acute asthma	• Pneumothorax • Fb • OSA • Kyphoscoliosis • Severe apnea • NM disorders • Exhaustion • CNS	• Post surgery • Acute pancreatitis • Septic shock • DIC • Pneumocystitis carnnni **Clinical picture :** -Cause -Severe RD ..cyanosis **Criteria for diagnosis:** -Diffuse bilateral fluffy infilterate -ALVEOLAR – ARTERIAL PO2 difference increased -Pul capillary wedge pressure <18

		-Pao2 to fio2 ratio <-200 regardless peep **Exclude** o PUL embolism o CHF o Pneumonia o Respiratory failure o pnemothorax atelectasis
Investigation		
-Pulse oximetry alterative to ABG -VQ mismatch	-Pulse oximetry not used -ABG -Ventilation defect	
Treatment		
-Supplemental O2 -Improve it But low PO2 for FIO2	-Supplemental O2 -Improve hypoxemia- -Low PO2 improved -Not improve hypercapnea **So assisted ventilation**	-No response to supp O2 -MV(increase peep)

10- ENT , AUDIOMETRY AND TYMPANOGRAM

Acute Otitis Media	Otitis Externa	Otitis Media With Effusion =Secretory =Glue Ear
-Common complication of NasoPhyrigitis	-Infection of outer ear canal	-Sequence of acute otitis media Especially if recurrent
Causative Agent		
-Viral **-Bacterial :**strept pneumonae	-Staph aureus -Pseudomonas	Fluid collecting behind the tympanic membrane within middle ear in absence of inflammation
Clinical Picture		
-Fever ,irritability **-Otoscope :** **Initially :** -TM: retracted **Later :** -TM : Red , congestion ,bulge ,decrease movement with air insufflations =immobile TM	-Pain on pulling pinna (Tenderness) -Creamy discharge -Post cervical LN -Uncomplicated = intact TM -Complicated = perforated TM	- inattension ,learning difficulities -No signs of acute infection **-Otoscope:** -TM : • Dull • Sluggish movement

-IF Perforation of ear drum = severe pain followed by sudden improvement		
Complication : **Most common complication :** Acute and chronic mastioditis **Causative agent :** staph aureus **Investigations:** -CBC,blood culture -Ct confirm diagnosis **Clinical picture :** -localized swelling -Protruded auricle ,fever and otalgia **Treatment :** -Immediate iv antibiotic and refere to ENT		
Treatment		
-regular antipyretics and analgesics with GP review in 48 hours	-Topical ofloxacin (**FOP**)	-Self limited -Watchful waiting

-Indication of antibiotics in acute Otitis Media :
 	
-Less than 6 months age
 	
-Less than 2 years with bilateral acute otitis media
 	
-All ages with severe acute otitis media
 	
   o Systemic unwellness
   o Persistent symptoms for 4 days or longer
   o Perforation and discharge
Antibiotics used :
 	
-High dose amoxycilin 90 ml /kg /day
 	
-Iv ceftriaxone in newborn (**AKP**)
		For three months
		
		Indication of tympanostomy :
		
		-Bilateral persistent OME with conductive hearning loss
		
		-Any risk of speech delay as cystic fibrosis, down syndrome ,cleft palate
		
		-Recurrent acute otitis media with OME at time of assessment

Acute Pharyngitis Acute Tonsillitis	Peritonsillar Abcess	Acute Bacterial Sinusitis
Causative Agent		
-Viral -Bacterial : GABHS	GABHS	-Strept pneumonae

Indication of tonsillectomy
 	
(referral criteria)
 	
-Recurrent tonsillitis
 	
   More than 5 episodes in(2) consecutive years
 	
   +
 	
Disabling episodes preventing normal functioning
 	
-One or two episodes of quinsy
 	
-Obstructive sleep apnea
 	
-Suspicious of other pathology as lymphoma
		-Ethmoiditis
		
		Most common in children
		
		Because it is the only sinus present at birth
		
		Its Most common complication is orbital cellulitis
		
		-Maxillary sinus
		
		Clinically important after 18 month
		
		-Frontal
		
		Complicated brain abcess at 8 years
		
		-spheniodal
		
		begin to develop after 6 years

Streptococcal pharyngitis : -Abrupt onset ->3 years old -High fever -sore throat -enlarged anterior cervical LN -no cough =tonsillitis -headache -abdominal pain -palatal petechae **differential diagnosis :** **viral pharyngitis :** rhinovirus: adenovirus : -High fever – Cough,coryza conjunctivitis - typically : follicular pharyngitis **Ebestein barr virus :** -Exudative	-High fever -Drooling -Dysphagia -Distress -Neck hyperextension **Signs :** -unilateral tonsillar swelling pushing uvula to contralateral side -Trismus -Reffered otalgia -Jugulo digastric ,cervical lymphadenopathy	**-Clinical** diagnosis rather than radiological diagnosis especially in children less than 6 years old **One of three will diagnose acute bacterial sinusitis :** -Persistent cough and nasal discharge more than 10 days without improvement -Fever more than 38,5 with purulent nasal discharge at least 3 days -Worsening of fever,cough and nasal discharge after 3-4 days period of improvement **Others :** -free chest examination -cough mostly early morning due to post nasal discharge

pharyngitis -fatigue		**Uncommon**
-palatal petechae – splenomegally		- facial pain
- cervical lymphadenopathy		-headache worsen by bending, cough, sneezing
-fever Not respond to antibiotics within 48hours		
So you should do EBV serology		
So ,		
Exudate is not specific for bacterial infection		

Investigations :		
RAST	**Needle drainage=gold standard =**diagnostic and therapeutic	**Skull Xray**
-Only done if overlapping symptoms as cough and abdominal pain	In trendelberg position	-False negative results are common
-done on pharyngeal secretion obtained by swab	-If fail to obtain pus indication for surgical incision	**CT :**gold standard especially if orbital involvement is suspected
-if result of RAST is negative ,second sample sent for GAS culture.		**Treatment :** Amoxicillin for 10 days

Orbital Cellulitis	Preseptal Cellulitis	Cavernous Sinus Thrombosis
-Staph aureas Risk factor : paranasal sinusitis (in 90% of patient) -Signs of systemic infection		
Unilateral		Bilateral
Not cross supraorbital ridge	Cross supraorbital ridge=swelling confined to eyelid	Meningism : triade of nuchal rigidity ,photophobia and headache
No cranial nerve involvement		-Cranial nerve 3 ,5 ,6 -Ptosis -Abscent corneal reflex -Lateral gaze palsy and diplopia
Vision normal early but later decrease visual acuity	Vision normal	Early vision loss
Painful restriction of extraoccular	No restriction of extraoccular	

movement (ophthalmoplegia)	movement	
Chemosis Red eye	No chemosis White globe	Chemosis
Proptosis	No proptosis	Proptosis
- ct orbit To exclude orbital abcess which need surgery **- ophthalmology refere**		**fundoscopy** -Papilledema -Dilated tortuous retinal vessels.
Immediate iv antibiotics Iv ceftriaxone (AKP)	-oral antibiotics	

Acase Of Preseptal Cellulitis

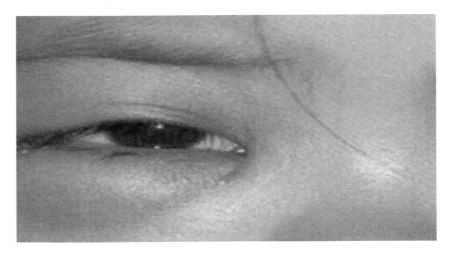

Acase Of Orbital Cellulitis

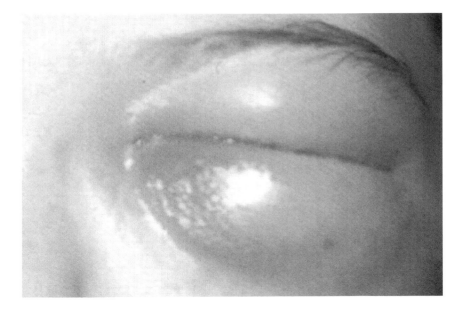

Obstructive Sleep Apnea	Allergic Rhinitis
-Upper airway collapse during sleep leading to apneas, nearly 30 apnea episodes of 10 sec ond duration or longer in 7 hours period secondary to airway obstruction	- type 1 hypersensitivity reaction -allergic conjunctivitis is present with more than 70 % of cases ,red itchy eye
-Occur During Rapid eye movement sleep	
-Type 2 respiratory failure =hypoxic hypercapnea	
-Peak 2-6 years	
-Boys=girls	
-No link to SIDS but premature death	
Risk factors : -Anatomic : obesity,large adenoid -Neurological : cerebral palsy	**Differential diagnosis :** -Adenoid hypertrophy -Nasopharyngitis -Vasomotor rhinitis

Clinical Picture	
-Mouth breathing ,snoring	**>one hour in most days of**
-Restlessness at sleep	-Sneezing
-Frequent awakening=decrease REM sleep	-nasal itching
	-Bilateral nasal obstruction=nasal speech
-Daytime hypersomnolence	
=narcolepsy .	-Bilateral watery nasal discharge
-road traffic accident	<ul><li>Long duration</li><li>Dramatic response to nasal decongestant</li><li>FH of atopy</li></ul>
-Early morning headache	
-Poor school performance	**Signs:**
-FTT	**-Allergic salute :**
-Pulmonary hypertension and core pulmonale	Transverse crease in lower nose
	-Allergic facies:
-Nocturnal enuresis	Open mouth ,midface hypoplasia
	-Allergic shiner :
	Dark puffy lower eye lid
	-Nasal polyp, if associated with growth failure ,
	-sweat test should be done to exclude cystic fibrosis
	-chest xray should be done to exclude dextrocardia
	-Pale or bluish mucous membrane of nose

Investigations	
-Polysomnography (Rarely available) -Replaced by nocturnal pulse oximetry =simple sleep study = gold standard for diagnosis -It is overnight monitoring of RR HR o2 saturation to exclude other causes of snorning .	**-Skin prick test** (of choice)**AKP** -indicated when etiology is unclear before arduous allergen avoidance . I.e house dust mite allergy should be confirmed before avoidance. - skin test better than igE
Treatment	
-Adenotonsillectomy - Not just adenoid - Done after confirmed diagnosis by polysomnography **-CPAP at night** **-**mainstay treatment in adult but limited in children -Done if contraindicated adenotonsillectomy **-Recently . LRA** **-Decrease weight** **-Avoid supine position**	**Intermittent :** -Topical antihistaminics (azelastine) **Persistant :** -Topical corticosteroids when nasal block or nasal polyp is primary complaint . **-Oral non sedating antihistamincs :** **Cetirizine** It is first line in the following situations : -conjunctivitis is present -2-5 years age -patient preference of oral treatment

AUDIMETRY INTERPRETATION

Hearing Impairement

- otitis media with effusion is most common cause in preschool,will be short term hearning affection

Steps Of Interpretations :

o **STEP 1**

- O for rt ear air conduction
- X for lt ear air conduction
- > or triangle for bone conduction

o **STEP 2 (RANGE OF HEARING)**

- 0-20 Db give normal speech perception
- 20-40 DB   normal speech is heared as whisper
- 40-60 DB   difficult to hear loud speech
- More than 60 DB   indicate profound loss of hearning

o **STEP 3 (TYPE OF HEARING LOSS)**

1. normal bone conduction + abnormal air conduction = conductive hearing loss
2. abnormal bone conduction + normal air conduction = sensorineural hearing loss
3. abnormal bone conduction + abnormal air conduction + gap between them < 10db = sensorineural hearing loss
4. abnormal bone conduction + abnormal air conduction + gap between them > 10db = mixed hearing
5. abnormal air conduction of mild degree 20-40 =conductive hearnng loss
6. abnormal air conduction of moderate or severe degree more than 40 = SNHL
7. high frequency loss of hearning = SNHL

Hearning Tests : AKP

- pure tone audiometry : for children 5 years and older
- behavioural observation audiometry : 6 months or older
- distraction test& visual reinforcement audiometry : between 7-30 months
- play audiometry : between 30month and 5 years

Management :

SNHL	CHL
-Affect cochlea in inner ear,auditory nerve -Bacterial meningitis = pure SNHL	-Affect outer and middle ear function
-bilateral cochlear implants better benefits than unilateral implants(not recommened by NICE guidelines) -optimum age : one year	

Audiogram showing bilateral mixed hearning loss

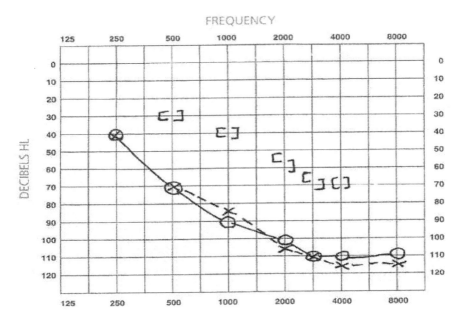

Acase of right conductive hearing loss

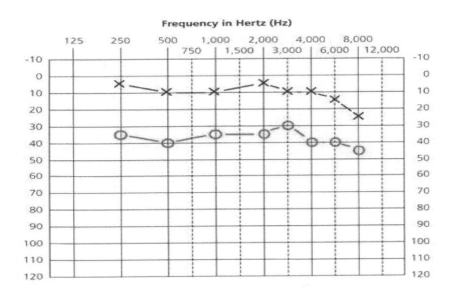

Tympanogram

- Sound probe placed in ear canal
- Changes in ear canal volume plotted against changes in pressure
- This give an indication of how well the eardrum moves in response to sound

1. abnormal high volme suggest perforated drum
2. flat curve suggest OME
3. shifting to left (peak at negative pressures)suggest eustacian tube obstruction (decrease compliance of tympanic membrane)

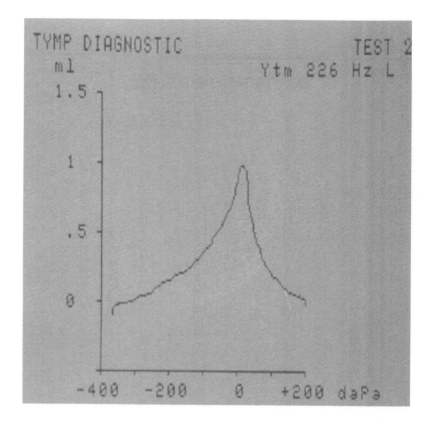

ABOUT THE AUTHOR

Dr Haitham Hassabou MBBS MRCPCH
Pediatrician And Neonatologist
Formly Pediatrician At BENCH Hospital
Tanta University Hospitals